HISTAMINE INTOLERANCE DIET

A Beginner's 3-Week Step-by-Step to Managing Histamine Intolerance with Recipes and Meal Plan

Brandon Gilta

mindplusfood

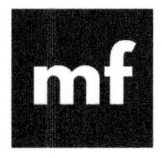

Copyright © 2020 Brandon Gilta

All rights reserved

No part of this book may be reproduced, or stored in a retrieval system, or transmitted in any form or by any means, electronic, mechanical, photocopying, recording, or otherwise, without express written permission of the publisher.

Printed in the United States of America

DISCLAIMER

By reading this disclaimer, you are accepting the terms of the disclaimer in full. If you disagree with this disclaimer, please do not read the guide.

All of the content within this guide is provided for informational and educational purposes only, and should not be accepted as independent medical or other professional advice. The author is not a doctor, physician, nurse, mental health provider, or registered nutritionist/dietician. Therefore, using and reading this guide does not establish any form of a physician-patient relationship.

Always consult with a physician or another qualified health provider with any issues or questions you might have regarding any sort of medical condition. Do not ever disregard any qualified professional medical advice or delay seeking that advice because of anything you have read in this guide. The information in this guide is not intended to be any sort of medical advice and should not be used in lieu of any medical advice by a licensed and qualified medical professional.

The information in this guide has been compiled from a variety of known sources. However, the author cannot attest to or guarantee the accuracy of each source and thus should not be held liable for any errors or omissions.

You acknowledge that the publisher of this guide will not be held liable for any loss or damage of any kind incurred as a result of this guide or the reliance on any information provided within this guide. You acknowledge and agree that you assume all risk and responsibility for any action you undertake in response to the information in this guide.

Using this guide does not guarantee any particular result (e.g., weight loss or a cure). By reading this guide, you acknowledge that there are no guarantees to any specific outcome or results you can expect.

All product names, diet plans, or names used in this guide are for identification purposes only and are the property of their respective owners. The use of these names does not imply endorsement. All other trademarks cited herein are the property of their respective owners.

Where applicable, this guide is not intended to be a substitute for the original work of this diet plan and is, at most, a supplement to the original work for this diet plan and never a direct substitute. This guide is a personal expression of the facts of that diet plan.

Where applicable, persons shown in the cover images are stock photography models and the publisher has obtained the rights to use the images through license agreements with third-party stock image companies.

CONTENTS

Title Page
Copyright
Disclaimer
Introduction — 1
All About Histamine — 3
Notes for the Histamine Intolerant — 10
A Potential 3-Step Guide on How to Get Started with Low-Histamine Diet — 16
Low-Histamine Diet — 18
How to Master the Low-Histamine Diet (Week 1) — 24
How to Create a Meal Plan (Week 2) — 27
How to Sustain the Low-Histamine Diet (Week 3) — 32
Sample Recipes — 34
Conclusion — 43
FAQ — 45
References and Helpful Links — 47

INTRODUCTION

According to several studies and research conducted, histamine intolerance happens to 1% of the world population—80% of which are of the middle-aged population group. However, because histamine intolerance is characterized by the same symptoms as common allergies, most physicians diagnose these intolerance cases as allergies. Hence, it is called a pseudo-allergy or "fake" allergy.

Histamine was discovered by Dale and Laidlaw in 1910. And in 1932, it was found to be a mediator of allergic reactions which may be deadly for some people with severe cases. Now, histamine is defined as a substance produced by our immune system which acts as a defense mechanism against external bodies that may harm you. It is also responsible for allergic reactions such as tearing up, sneezing, and itching. Hence, the production of antihistamines stops these allergic reactions for the comfort of people with allergies.

However, histamine levels in your body may rise, which may result in fluctuating blood pressure, disturbances to your heart rhythm, and neurological pathway disturbances. This condition is known as histamine intolerance—which may be fatal because histamine intolerance, as mentioned earlier in the text, is commonly misdiagnosed with other allergies. Thus, the patients are not given the proper treatments for histamine intolerance.

Enteral histaminosis, commonly known as histamine intolerance, is a condition in which a person is sensitive to histamine-containing foods. It is a condition that has been just discovered this century and is associated with the inability to break down dietary histamine.

Histamine is only known as a chemical made by our bodies that is responsible for protecting our bodies from life-threatening allergens. But most people do not know that even foods and drinks contain histamine. So, this guide is made for people who have or may have internal histaminosis. We will help you to know what your condition is and how to cope with it through the histamine intolerance diet. After reading this guide, you will be able to answer the following questions:
- What is histamine intolerance?
- What are its symptoms?
- How it develops
- How to know if you are histamine intolerant
- What lifestyle changes do you need to do if you are histamine intolerant?
- What food and drinks do you need to watch out for

Check it out!

ALL ABOUT HISTAMINE

What Is Histamine?
Histamine is a neurotransmitter and hormone produced in the body that serves many important functions. It plays a key role in our body's immune response, mediating allergic reactions, maintaining healthy energy and blood flow levels, and promoting ample digestion. Histamine also has a psychotropic component; when we are feeling good or under stress, histamine helps to convey our emotional state.

Histamine plays an important role in regulating the body's inflammatory response. When foreign invaders enter the body, such as allergens or antigens, histamine is released into the bloodstream from mast cells or basophils. This triggers an inflammatory response which can include symptoms like redness and swelling of tissues, itching, and difficulty breathing due to constricted airways. Histamine works with other immune system cells to fight off these invaders and protect us from harm.

Histamine is also involved in autoimmune disorders such as allergies or asthma, where it is released inappropriately by the body's immune system resulting in overactive inflammatory responses. In such cases, antihistamines are used to reduce inflammation by blocking the action of histamine on its receptors throughout the body.

Histamines play a key role in keeping energy levels balanced by helping to regulate how much glucose (sugar) enters the bloodstream after meals. They can keep appetite under control while controlling satiety signals to ensure we aren't overeating. When there is excess sugar circulating in our bloodstream they act as a brake on this process causing it to slow down temporarily until insulin can help manage it more efficiently.

Histamines are necessary for healthy blood circulation as they act as vasodilators promoting better blood flow throughout our bodies so that oxygenated blood can reach all parts of us more easily including vital organs like our brain and heart which require adequate amounts of oxygenated blood for proper functioning.

Finally, histamines are key players in promoting healthy digestion by stimulating stomach acid production thus allowing proteins to be broken down into smaller molecules so that our bodies will be able to absorb nutritious vitamins and minerals found within them more effectively. Histamines also trigger contractions within digestive muscles aiding food transit through all stages of digestion from mouth to anus.

What Is Histamine Intolerance?
Histamine intolerance is a condition caused by an unbalanced level of histamine in the body. Histamine is a naturally occurring chemical found in many foods, as well as within our bodies. When the amount of histamine in our bodies is too high, usually due to inefficient metabolism, it can create unpleasant symptoms such as headaches and nasal congestion.

The main cause of histamine intolerance is an inherited deficiency or absence of the enzyme diamine oxidase (DAO). DAO breaks down dietary histamine and helps keep levels from reaching toxic levels in the body. Without sufficient DAO, histamine levels build up more quickly and symptoms begin to appear when consuming certain foods high in histamine.

Imbalances in other enzymes involved in regulating histamines may also play a role. Histamines are normally broken down by monoamine oxidase A (MAOA) and B (MAOB) enzymes. If the MAOA and MAOB enzymes are lower than normal, they won't be able to process all of the extra histamines in your system. This means that more free-floating histamines will remain active longer in your bloodstream, causing your typical symptoms associated with allergies or sensitivities such as fatigue, digestive issues, skin rashes, and more.

In addition to genetic predisposition for lower levels of DAO or MAOA/B enzymes, many environmental factors can contribute to increased levels of histamines including exposure to environmental allergens like dust mites or mold; stress; alcohol consumption; certain medications such as pain killers; smoking; and certain illnesses like mastocytosis where immune cells release higher amounts of histamine into circulation.

All these triggers lead to heightened sensitivity towards things high in this natural biochemical compound that can cause an allergy-like reaction even if no allergic response has been established before consuming them.

In summary, people with a hereditary deficiency or absence of the enzyme DAO are often at risk for developing an intolerance to dietary sources of histamine due to their inability to efficiently break down this attributed biochemical compound effectively leading to imbalances within the body which can create further sensitivities when exposed to other external or internal factors making one predisposed to experiencing typical allergens-associated reactions even without any prior allergic reaction experienced beforehand.

What Are Its Symptoms?

Histamine intolerance is a condition characterized by an inability to break down histamines, which can lead to a variety of uncomfortable symptoms. Here are 10 common symptoms associated with histamine intolerance:

Skin rash or hives: Histamine intolerance can be indicated by an itchy, red skin rash or hives. It is usually indicated by a raised area on the skin along with slight swelling and itching. These symptoms can be found anywhere on the body, making the individual highly uncomfortable.

Headaches: Individuals who experience histamine intolerance may also suffer from headaches. The intensity of the pain associated with these headaches can vary, but in many cases, they can be quite severe. In particular, it is common for people with histamine intolerance to report experiencing more discomfort or even intensified headache pain when consuming certain foods or drinking alcohol. As such, it is important for those who are affected by histamine intolerance to remain aware of potential triggers and practice moderation to minimize headache symptoms.

Nausea: Symptoms of histamine intolerance vary in severity and frequency, but one of the most common symptoms is nausea. Those dealing with this condition may experience queasiness after consuming high-histamine foods or drinks. In addition to nausea, abdominal cramping, and bloating are often experienced by those who have histamine intolerance.

Diarrhea: Diarrhea can occur due to histamine intolerance as well, primarily when high-histamine food or beverages are consumed. It may also be accompanied by stomach cramps and feverishness.

Fatigue: Fatigue is a particularly common sign, appearing suddenly after consuming certain foods or drinks that contain high levels of histamine. To help address fatigue, resting and drinking hydrating fluids are beneficial. In many cases, this helps return energy fairly quickly; however, for those who don't take steps soon enough, the fatigue may persist for hours.

Flushing: A symptom of histamine intolerance that is often seen by those affected is flushing. This commonly involves the reddening of the facial and neck area as a result of elevated levels of histamines in the bloodstream, but can equally be integrated with other symptoms such as headaches or skin rashes. Those afflicted with this condition should make sure to identify and manage their triggers, whatever they may be, to help limit their exposure.

Heart palpitations: After eating foods or beverages that are high in histamines, those who struggle to metabolize these compounds could experience heart palpitations or arrhythmia. This can drastically alter an individual's normal heartbeat and cause long-term issues such as fatigue, anxiousness, and related physical symptoms depending on the person's level of sensitivity. It is important to seek help from a medical professional if these signs appear.

Congestion and wheezing: Histamine intolerance manifests in different ways depending on the individual, but two symptoms that are commonly experienced by those with histamine intolerance are congestion and wheezing. This occurs when there is an inflammation of the airways due to increased amounts of histamines, which are natural chemicals that certain foods contain. People with histamine intolerance may notice that nasal congestion and wheezing occur more frequently after eating certain foods, indicating to them which foods should be avoided to reduce discomfort related to histamine intolerance.

Insomnia: One common symptom associated with Histamine Intolerance is insomnia, as higher levels of histamines lead to greater difficulty in falling asleep and staying asleep. Many people struggle to function at their best when suffering from this type of sleep deprivation due to its negative impact on cognitive performance. In addition, insomnia can be a symptom of other underlying issues, so if you are experiencing difficulty sleeping it's important to visit your doctor for testing and rule out any other underlying factors that could be contributing. Ultimately, diagnosing and addressing histamine intolerance can go a long way toward achieving optimal health.

Mood swings: Histamine intolerance can cause several physical symptoms that vary in severity. One of the most common and uncommonly noted symptoms is mood swings. When histamines accumulate in the body, these chemical responses can lead to sudden changes in one's emotional state, being that they are both inflammatory and excitatory substances. This occurrence can be fleeting or even chronic in some cases, depending on the strength of the response as well as various other factors at play.

If you're experiencing any of the symptoms listed, it's important to seek help from a trained medical professional. Histamine intolerance can lead to serious health problems if left untreated, and early intervention is key in managing your condition. Following an appropriate diet is one way that you can effectively manage histamine intolerance and limit its effects.

Is Histamine the Same As Food Allergies?
Histamine intolerance and food allergies are two conditions often confused with one another. While both reactions can be triggered by the ingestion of certain substances, their underlying mechanisms, symptoms, and treatments vary greatly.

Histamine intolerance is a condition characterized by an inability to properly break down histamines in foods. This results in a build-up of the chemical leading to numerous physical symptoms such as diarrhea, skin rashes, nausea, headache, and fatigue. In some cases, it can even lead to cardiovascular complications. Histamine intolerance is typically caused by low levels of diamine oxidase (DAO), which is an enzyme needed to metabolize histamines from food sources.

Food allergies are much more severe reactions that occur when the body perceives a particular substance as foreign or dangerous and the immune system responds aggressively by releasing chemicals such as histamines. The reaction can range from mild to life-threatening depending on how prone someone is to allergies. Symptoms of food allergies include hives, swelling, difficulty breathing, and vomiting. Unlike histamine intolerance, these reactions are caused by an antibody IgE which recognizes and binds to the protein in food that it deems foreign or dangerous and triggers the response of releasing histamines.

The main challenge when dealing with either condition is detecting what triggered the reaction. Determining whether someone has histamine intolerance or an allergy requires additional testing such as skin prick tests for IgE antibodies to accurately diagnose their condition before beginning any treatment plan. Unfortunately due to the similarity between their underlying mechanisms, these conditions are often misdiagnosed which can hinder future treatment plans and lead to complications if undetected initially.

NOTES FOR THE HISTAMINE INTOLERANT

Diagnosis

The normal histamine levels of a person should only be from 0.3 ng/mL to 1.0 ng/mL. If you exceed this, you may experience the symptoms mentioned in the previous part after ingesting histamine-rich foods. But, until now, there are still no clear clinical signs and symptoms that would sure-fire diagnose histamine intolerance.

To diagnose a histamine intolerance case, it is recommended that the patient should have at least two of the mentioned symptoms above before rendering an official diagnosis. The physician must also require the patient to keep track of his/her food intake along with the symptoms that he/she might experience upon eating the food suspected to be the reason for the symptoms. This allows a thorough examination of the relationship between the patient's food intake with the symptoms.

Then, the doctor will try to eliminate some food that may be the cause of the symptoms. If proven related, then the patient is declared histamine intolerant.

Another test that was proposed to diagnose histamine intolerance would be the prick test; wherein the physician pricks the patient somewhere in his/her body and applies 1% histamine solution on the pricked area. This is based on a study conducted in 2011, wherein the subjects were made to undergo the same procedure as mentioned. It turned out with a 79% positive, the people with suspected histamine intolerance were revealed to have a small itchy, red bump on the pricked area that did not tone down within 50 minutes.

Lastly, the doctor may need to get your blood sample to know if you have DAO (diamine oxidase) efficiency because this enzyme is responsible for breaking down histamine. Abnormal DAO levels indicate histamine intolerance. Also, DAO levels in the body are affected by excessive alcohol intake and drug use.

Treatments

Histamine intolerance is a condition where the body is unable to process excessive levels of histamine in the bloodstream. Medical treatments for this condition include avoiding foods that are high in histamine, taking antihistamines, and using probiotics, among other treatments.

Avoiding foods high in histamine: The first step to treating histamine intolerance is avoiding foods that are high in histamine. This includes foods like fermented dairy products, certain fish and seafood, processed meats, pickles, tomatoes, spinach, and other vegetables. In addition to these many people with histamine intolerance have sensitivities or allergies to specific foods such as citrus fruits and nuts. Those with this condition need to be aware of what they should avoid so that they don't trigger an uncomfortable reaction.

Antihistamines: Another common treatment for histamine intolerance is taking antihistamines. These medications block the action of the chemical called histamine which is responsible for causing many of the symptoms associated with histamine intolerance such as skin rashes, headaches, and nausea. Antihistamines can also be used to treat allergic reactions caused by sensitivity to particular allergens such as pet dander or pollen. They typically come in pill form and are taken orally regularly or as needed when a reaction occurs.

Probiotics: Probiotics are live microorganisms that can be found naturally in certain foods like yogurt or fermented vegetables as well as dietary supplements available over-the-counter at most pharmacies or health food stores. Probiotics have been shown to help reduce inflammation in the digestive system which can help alleviate some of the uncomfortable symptoms associated with histamine intolerance including abdominal pain, bloating, and gas.

Vitamin C: Increasing your intake of vitamin C may also be beneficial in treating this condition as it's been shown to reduce levels of circulating histamines in the body which can help alleviate symptoms associated with an adverse reaction due to this condition. Vitamin C supplements may be taken orally daily but it's important to keep in mind that consuming too much vitamin C has been linked to side effects like gastrointestinal upset so it's best not to exceed the recommended dosage without first consulting your doctor.

Immunoglobulin Replacement Therapy (IGRT): Intravenous Immunoglobulin Replacement Therapy (IGRT) is a relatively new medical procedure that seeks to address some of the more unpleasant physical symptoms of histamine disorders like allergies. It's administered by trained healthcare practitioners and consists of infusions of healthy antibodies, designed to reduce circulating levels of histamines while also boosting immunity against future episodes. Properly managed over a course of time by specialists such as allergists/immunologists, IGRT can be highly beneficial in mitigating the effects of such ailments and has been officially sanctioned via various regulatory agencies, thus making it widely accessible to the public.

Complications

Histamine intolerance is a condition that results from an increase of histamine in the body. The severe symptoms of histamine intolerance can include digestive issues, skin rashes, migraine headaches, and respiratory problems.

Digestive issues: Histamines are a molecule that the body typically releases as part of the immune response to allergens and other irritants. Unfortunately, those who suffer from histamine intolerance can experience an over-release of histamine which leads to a range of nasty digestive issues. These can include abdominal pain, cramping, bloating, gas, diarrhea, and constipation - none of which are enjoyable. Fortunately, there are treatments available that help to reduce histamine production and thereby lessen the symptoms related to histamine intolerance.

Skin rashes: Histamine reactions are known to increase inflammation in the body and may cause the skin to react with rashes, itching, and hives. When histamine levels become too high, this can lead to hives (urticaria), which is when red or pale bumps appear on the surface of the skin. Histamines may also irritate eczema-affected skin, leading to a similar itchy, inflamed rash that can be difficult to treat.

While antihistamines are often used to reduce symptoms of excess histamine release, long-term management of these bothersome skin rashes requires an evaluation by a dermatologist to identify the root cause of the reaction.

Migraine and headaches: For those living with histamine intolerance, the potential for migraines is a constant threat. Diagnosed through food and symptom tracking, migraine headaches caused by histamines in specific foods can cause intense physical pain and disability that can last for hours or even days. Fortunately, the range of dietary changes available to those suffering from histamine intolerance can help mitigate the risks of these debilitating migraines, allowing them to live full lives without compromising their health.

Respiratory problems: Asthma is a condition that can cause serious respiratory problems if not addressed. High levels of histamines, which can be triggered by exposure to certain allergens or heat, can exacerbate these symptoms, resulting in coughing, wheezing, and shortness of breath. Unfortunately, though asthma is a common problem, preventing or treating respiratory difficulties due to histamine sensitivity can be challenging.

Allergy medications and environmental controls may help mitigate the impact of histamine levels on the lungs and surrounding structures. In addition to medical intervention, breathing techniques may encourage lung expansion and help open the airways for easier breathing; however, it is best to talk to your doctor before trying any new methods as severe cases may need immediate attention.

Nausea and vomiting: Histamine has several important regulatory functions in the body, such as regulating the immune response and helping with digestion. However, when too much histamine is produced, it can cause symptoms that disrupt normal digestion processes, leading to nausea and vomiting. Research suggests that this can occur when Histamine-2 receptor antagonists are taken to reduce stomach acid production in the stomach or intestines.

Additionally, several other medical conditions can contribute to excess histamine levels which may lead to nausea and vomiting. It is important to consult with a doctor if symptoms persist; they will be able to help identify a potential underlying cause of your nausea and vomiting that can be treated accordingly.

Anaphylaxis: Anaphylaxis is a potentially life-threatening allergic reaction that can be triggered by high histamine levels. This severe reaction can cause swelling, difficulty breathing, and even shock if not immediately treated with an epinephrine injection (epi-pen).

Everyone should keep a close eye on the histamine levels in their bodies, especially if they are prone to severe allergic reactions or have medical allergies. Clinical symptoms of anaphylaxis can begin to manifest within minutes of exposure and require emergency medical attention. Understanding the ways one might trigger anaphylaxis is essential for all individuals to keep themselves safe and healthy.

Difficulty sleeping: Studies have shown that for those who have histamine intolerance, difficulty sleeping can become a common problem. Rapid fluctuations in blood sugar levels due to high levels of histamines present in certain foods can set off runaway adrenaline, leading to drowsiness during the daytime hours and an inability to fully rest at night.

As the night progresses, these individuals may find themselves wide awake and unable to sleep properly. This can result in unsatisfactory or no sleep during any given night period. As such, sufferers of histamine intolerance are encouraged to pay close attention to diet and accordingly avoid food that could trigger difficulty falling asleep or staying asleep throughout the night.

Anxiety/fatigue/brain fog: People who suffer from anxiety, fatigue, and brain fog may not know the connection to high levels of histamines. Histamines are a natural chemical produced in the body to provide a line of defense against invading pathogens and irritants. They are released by mast cells as part of an immune system response.

However, when excess amounts occur, it can cause excessive inflammation and allergic reactions which contribute to anxiety, fatigue, and mental confusion. It is important for those suffering from these conditions to discuss ways to monitor their histamine levels with their doctor to properly address their symptoms.

A POTENTIAL 3-STEP GUIDE ON HOW TO GET STARTED WITH LOW-HISTAMINE DIET

The Low-Histamine Diet is a useful method for alleviating the symptoms that are often brought on by a wide variety of food allergies and intolerances. It might be beneficial to have a strategy in place before beginning this type of nutritional approach if you are interested in getting started with it. The following are the first three actions that you should do to get started on the Low-Histamine Diet:

Step 1: Familiarize yourself with the basics
Before beginning any kind of diet, it is essential to have a solid understanding of what the diet involves and the reasoning behind why it is effective. Get familiar with the scientific underpinning of this approach to dieting, including what histamine intolerance is and how following a diet low in histamine can help lessen the symptoms associated with allergies and other types of intolerances.

Step 2: Eliminate high-histamine foods

To successfully adhere to a diet low in histamine, you will need to remove specific dietary triggers entirely, or at the least, severely restrict your consumption of them. To get started, eliminate the foods that contribute the most to your problem from your regular diet.

Aged meat, processed meats, fermented dairy products (like yogurt), fermented vegetables (like sauerkraut and kimchi), canned fish, aged cheeses, ripe fruits and vegetables, beer, wine, and spirits, as well as many sauces and condiments like ketchup or miso paste, are examples of common foods that are high in histamines. If you discover that eating certain meals causes negative reactions in your body after eating them, you may wish to restrict your consumption of such foods or consume them in only modest quantities.

Step 3: Introduce new food sources
If you want to effectively follow the low-histamine diet, the first thing you need to do is get rid of particular foods that are known to be triggers for your condition. However, adding new things to your routine may be just as useful. It is best to reintroduce foods high in tyramine, which plays an important role in the decomposition of histamines, into your diet gradually so that your body has time to readjust (e.g., bananas or salmon). Additionally, several herbs have been shown to reduce the effects of histamine; if you want to reap the benefits of these herbs throughout the day, search for dishes that include turmeric or ginger.

By understanding the basics of the Low-Histamine Diet and carefully incorporating new practices into your routine, you can make a smooth transition to this dietary approach. With time and patience, you may find that many of your symptoms (related to allergies or intolerances) start to diminish, allowing you to live more comfortably.

LOW-HISTAMINE DIET

A low-histamine diet is a dietary plan that avoids foods with high levels of histamine, which is a compound found in many foods. The main principles of the low-histamine diet are to limit or eliminate all sources of histamine-containing foods or foods that trigger the release of histamines. Additionally, certain supplements may need to be taken to ensure proper detoxification pathways and adequate nutrient intake.

The low-histamine diet is typically recommended for people who suffer from an allergy or intolerance to histamine-containing foods, such as those with Histamine Intolerance (HIT) or mast cell activation syndromes (MCAS). These individuals often present with symptoms such as headaches, digestive problems, chronic fatigue, mood disorders, and skin reactions after ingesting high-histamine foods. By avoiding those specific foods, their symptoms may be reduced significantly.

Low-histamine diets should also address any underlying issues that cause the body to have difficulty breaking down the natural histamines in food. It is important to note that these diets do not need to be overly restrictive to be effective—patients can still enjoy a wide variety of fresh produce while avoiding problem foods. Additionally, patients need to work with a qualified healthcare practitioner when starting this type of diet so they can monitor progress and adjust as needed.

Foods to Limit or Eliminate
- beer, champagne, and wine
- canned tuna, mackerel, sardines
- dried fruit products
- eggplant, spinach, tomatoes, avocados, spinach
- legumes
- miso, soy sauce, tempeh, and other fermented soy products
- pickles, kimchi, sauerkraut, and other fermented vegetables
- processed and takeout food
- salami, ham, sausages, and other fermented or cured meat
- shellfish
- sourdough
- yogurt, sour cream, aged cheese, and other fermented dairy products

You might notice that most food products high in histamine are fermented. This is because these foods contain bacteria that may live in the gut, prompting the body to make more histamine to fight these bacteria off.

On the other hand, the next list is made up of food items that may trigger the production or release of histamine in the body. The following foods are:
- alcohol
- bananas
- beans
- cashews, peanuts, walnuts, and other nuts
- chocolate and cocoa
- citrus fruits
- food additives
- food dye
- papaya
- preservatives
- tomatoes
- wheat germ

Lastly, this list contains different food items that block the enzyme DAO, thus, slowing down the breakdown of histamine:
- a couple of yogurt types—depending on the bacteria in it
- alcohol
- energy drink
- green tea, mate tea, black tea
- pineapple, kiwi, strawberries
- raw eggs

There may seem to be A LOT to avoid. Fortunately, histamine-rich foods are not a one-time-eat close to disaster. To have high levels of histamine, it takes several servings before you experience the symptoms.

For example, a bite or two of pineapples as breakfast dessert may be fine but having a ham and cheese sandwich for lunch may not be ideal.

Remember that the key is to limit, and not to exclude.

Besides, most histamine-rich foods have high levels of nutrients that are beneficial to us. So, hang in there and plan your meals properly to still get optimal nutrition.

Recommended Foods to Consume
Speaking of planning meals, you may be curious about what kind of foods may be consumed in this type of diet. Therefore, here is a list to keep you motivated:
- chicken
- cooking oil like olive oil
- cream cheeses, butter
- fresh fish
- fresh fruits except for plantains
- fresh meat
- fresh milk
- fresh vegetables (except the ones listed above) like carrots, cucumber, zucchini, celery, and shallots

- fruit juice except for citrus ones
- green leafy vegetables except for spinach
- herbal tea except the ones mentioned above
- herbs
- quinoa, rice, almond milk, coconut milk, and other gluten-free fruit
- whole grains like bread, crackers, pasta, and noodles

Contrary to those excluded from the diet, these foods included generally fresh and organic foods. This is because less processing has been done to them.

The Benefits of a Low-Histamine Diet

A low-histamine diet is beneficial for individuals who suffer from histamine intolerance. This type of diet involves removing foods that contain high amounts of histamine and replacing them with safe, histamine-low choices. Here are 8 benefits of following a low-histamine diet:

Lower allergic reactions: One major benefit of a low-histamine diet is the ability to reduce allergic reactions triggered by histamines. Removing common triggers like fermented foods and aged products can help reduce symptoms caused by allergies and intolerances.

Improved digestive health: By eliminating foods that are high in histamines, individuals can improve their digestive health since the body will not have to work as hard to process foods that it is unable to tolerate well. A lower intake of histamines can also help prevent other digestive issues, such as bloating and abdominal pain.

Reduced headaches and migraines: High levels of histamines have been linked to increased headaches and migraines in some individuals. Following a low-histamine diet can reduce these issues by helping the body maintain properly balanced levels of histamines in the bloodstream and reducing inflammation in the brain's pathways.

Improved mood and energy levels: Eating a healthy low-histamine diet may help to increase energy levels in some people by providing sustained energy rather than short bursts caused by eating highly processed or sugary snacks that are rich in histamines. As an added benefit, because fewer allergens are being introduced into the body when problem foods are cut out, there is less chance for mood swings or distress reactions due to high amounts of histamines present in the bloodstream.

Better hormonal balance: When the body has higher concentrations of hormones like estrogen or progesterone present due to food intolerances, this can throw off natural hormone balances leading to problems like premenstrual syndrome (PMS) or premenstrual dysphoric disorder (PMDD). Following a low-histamine diet helps reduce these issues since cutting out many food triggers helps balance out hormones over time as they adjust more naturally in response to lower levels of exposure to problem foods and irritants present in high doses within them.

Increased nutrient absorption: Food sensitivities like those seen with intolerances or allergies can decrease nutrient absorption from our diets. This is because our bodies may reject particular nutrients present within specific ingredients or meals. However, a low-histamine diet helps ensure that there is higher nutrient uptake since fewer allergens are being introduced into our systems at any one time. This makes the digestion process easier on our bodies overall resulting in better absorption rates for each meal we take in each day!

Better skin health: Many individuals with allergies may experience skin irritation due to their sensitivity to certain substances found within food items. However, cutting them out through following dietary restrictions such as a low-histamine diet can allow skin conditions such as eczema or rashes to improve over time. This becomes more effective if properly managed with other lifestyle changes as well including proper hydration strategies and stress management tactics!

Safer fertility options: While links between food sensitivities/allergies and infertility still need further study, keeping lower amounts of problem substances within your diets may help those looking for safer fertility options since ingesting too much allergen material could potentially create an unfavorable environment for conception due to its effects on hormones or general wellness when left unchecked!

HOW TO MASTER THE LOW-HISTAMINE DIET (WEEK 1)

You already know what to eat and what not to eat. But each list may seem too overwhelming to memorize. So, here are general pointers to remember when starting the low-histamine diet, along with lifestyle habits that you may want to start.

Avoid or limit your intake of instant and processed foods. These kinds of food are heavily loaded with histamine as these foods contain preservatives, additives, and even dyes. These are also the ones that contain too much sodium. So, they are generally not good for the heart, and not good for the gut. Examples of these foods are canned ready-to-eat meals and even fast food.

Limit or avoid the intake of fermented food. As mentioned earlier, these kinds of food contain bacteria that prompt the immune system to release histamine to fight off these bacteria. So, more fermented food means more bacteria. And more bacteria mean more histamine! Examples of these foods are alcohol, cheese, yeast products, and stale food items.

Eat fresh foods as much as possible. Since we want fewer bacteria that will challenge histamine, we want our diet to consist of fresh food. Of course, you cannot always make sure that the food you buy is freshly cut, freshly caught, and newly harvested—frozen foods will do—as long as there are little to no preservatives added to them.

Consume organic products. Organic products are the freshest and most natural products out there that contain no preservatives. Although they spoil faster, it is guaranteed to be safe and healthy because they are raised or grown naturally.

Avoid alcohol intake. Although it is a staple of most parties and gatherings, alcohol is high in histamine. So, it is only right to limit or avoid alcohol. Not only that it is high in histamine. They may also give more work to your liver if taken excessively.

Learn how to cook. Since most foods have histamine, you cannot avoid them in your diet. And there may be little to no restaurants that have a low-histamine diet menu prepared for their guests, so why not learn to cook your own? In this way, you can control your portions, and monitor your histamine intake. It may be a daunting task, but you will get a hang of it soon! Just take it little by little and start with the basics.

Know your nutrient needs. Cutting out or limiting food means that you are cutting certain nutrients from your body. And these nutrients may even help you alleviate symptoms or improve the production of the DAO enzyme. Examples are vitamin B6, vitamin C, copper, manganese, and zinc which help in enhancing the ability of the DAO enzyme to break down histamine.

Consult a doctor or a dietitian. Specific diets like the low-histamine diet are just general diets for people with the same condition. These are helpful but consulting a doctor or a dietitian to have a personal diet plan specific to your physique, medical history, and food preferences, is still the best option. Since you will be cutting out foods that are high in nutrients, it is only proper to consult them to make sure that you are meeting your daily nutrient needs.

By following these pointers and lifestyle habits, you will make sure that your body is getting the most nutrition out of every meal.

HOW TO CREATE A MEAL PLAN (WEEK 2)

At this point, you are expected to have some of the pointers already etched on your mind. Therefore, it is time to help you with meal planning. To get you started, here is a sample 7-day meal plan.

Monday	Breakfast Egg sandwich in gluten-free bread AM Snack Sliced apples Lunch Salad greens with gluten-free croutons PM Snack Peeled pears Dinner Roast salmon and mixed vegetables (zucchini, carrot, and potatoes)
Tuesday	Breakfast Boiled egg (limit one egg for a day) and gluten-free toast AM Snack Sliced fresh bananas, diced fruits, and fruit syrups Lunch Grilled fresh chicken salad with vegetable greens PM Snack Trail mix Dinner Stirred-fried turkey with vegetables

Wednesday	Breakfast Peanut butter toast AM Snack Chia seeds with mixed fruits Lunch Chicken fajitas with gluten-free tortilla PM Snack Sunflower seeds Dinner Pork and beans
Thursday	Breakfast Almond milk and trail mix AM Snack Sliced kiwi, apple, and grape salad Lunch Grilled Chicken Salad PM Snack Fruit juice Dinner Skillet-pan free-range meat in olive oil with mixed vegetables

Friday	Breakfast Kale Fried Rice AM Snack Macadamia nuts Lunch Chicken stir fry PM Snack Fruit salad Dinner Stirred-fried chicken with vegetables
Saturday	Breakfast Egg on toast AM Snack Coleslaw Lunch Pad Thai with Chicken PM Snack Freshly sliced bananas Dinner Garlic Hummus
Sunday	Breakfast Coleslaw AM Snack Fruit salad Lunch Stir-fried Cabbages and Apples PM Snack Trail nuts Dinner Sweet Potato Soup

Another tip is to know your alternatives! Know what you are going to get if you run out of almond milk, nuts, butter, and gluten-free bread. In this way, you will have a variety of options for your meals.

HOW TO SUSTAIN THE LOW-HISTAMINE DIET (WEEK 3)

You already have your tips. You already have your meal plan. But how can you last longer in this lifestyle? Below are tips that can get you to start moving and will help keep you going.

<u>Practice discipline</u>. The key to having a successful lifestyle change like a diet is to make yourself disciplined enough to sustain this lifestyle. Be used to your new habits. Always keep in mind your goal. And do not get tempted easily.

<u>Keep a food diary</u>. The low-histamine diet is not just a diet that you are bound to keep forever. This diet is also designed to slowly help and train your stomach to ingest histamine-rich foods. By the time your symptoms have toned down, reintroducing histamine-loaded foods little by little is a part of this therapy too. So, keep a food diary and record what foods you can already tolerate, and what you can work on. This also helps in monitoring your progress.

<u>Introduce histamine-rich foods at the discretion of a professional</u>. About the previous tip, reintroducing histamine-rich foods is a

part of maintaining this diet. Make sure that you are supervised by a professional such as a doctor or a dietitian to keep yourself from overdoing this process.

Think of the long-term benefits. It may be difficult to start and thinking about all your favorite foods being left in the grocery aisle instead of adding them to your cart may be a bit nerve-wracking and tempting. But at the end of the day, this is all for yourself. If you continue the low-histamine diet with little to no symptoms, you might start eating your favorites again—even the histamine-rich ones.

Enjoy the diet. Nothing is more discouraging than doing something you do not like. The main takeaway from dieting is to enjoy it. It may have removed a lot of foods from your list but look at what is left. Be creative. You might even try new foods that are low in histamine and enjoy them. Also, eat what you truly want.

Now, we think you are ready to start this journey! To help you decide what meal to eat now, the next section is dedicated to some of the recipes that are included in the sample 7-day meal plan.

Bon Appetit!

SAMPLE RECIPES

Garlic Hummus

Ingredients:
- 12 heads of garlic, roasted
- 2 tsp. virgin coconut oil
- 2 12-cup muffin tins
- extra trays of ice cube

Instructions:
1. Preheat the oven to 400°F.
2. Cut off the top of each garlic head to make the top of the cloves visible.
3. Put each garlic head in a muffin tin cup.
4. Rub the top of the garlic heads with coconut oil.
5. Use the second muffin tin to cover the first one.
6. Put in the oven and wait for 30 minutes to bake.
7. Take the garlic cloves out of the heads.
8. You may place 4-5 cloves of garlic in each ice cube tray section to store leftovers.
9. Use olive oil to cover cloves and freeze.
10. Squeeze the frozen roasted garlic cubes out of the trays and store them using a container.

Coleslaw

Ingredients:
- 1/2 cup virgin olive oil
- 1/2 head of red cabbage, chopped into small pieces
- 1 head of green cabbage, chopped into small pieces
- 1 tsp. unrefined sea salt, finely ground
- 2 green onions, chopped
- 4 drops organic stevia
- 8 organic carrots, shredded
- optional: a bunch of cilantro, chopped
- optional: 1 green apple, chopped finely

Instructions:
1. Mix all the chopped vegetables.
2. Blend in salt, virgin olive oil, and stevia together using a whisk or a blender.
3. Pour the blended slaw into the mixed vegetables.
4. Add apples upon serving.

Sweet Potato Soup

Ingredients:
- 1 fennel bulb, chopped
- 1 fresh ginger, chopped into an inch
- 1 red onion, chopped
- 1 small fresh turmeric root, chopped
- 10 oz. frozen sweet potato cubes
- 12 oz. frozen cauliflower florets
- 2 cloves garlic, chopped
- black pepper
- sea salt
- fresh herbs, chopped
- water or 4 cups of veggie broth

Instructions:
1. Use a stovetop soup pot to combine all ingredients.
2. Boil the ingredients and simmer for 30 minutes until vegetables are tender and flavors have soaked into the broth.
3. Transfer the ingredients, by batch, into a blender. To achieve a chunkier soup, pulse a few times or blend to purée.
4. Top with fresh green herbs when served.

Pad Thai with Chicken

Ingredients:
- 1 lb. chicken breast tenderloins, cut into chunks
- pure sesame oil, to taste
- 1 cup thinly sliced carrots
- 1/2 cup white mushrooms, chopped
- 1/2 bag of frozen pepper and onions blend, thawed
- 2 cloves of garlic, finely chopped
- 1/2 cup Egg Beaters
- 8 oz. zucchini noodles
- 2 tsp. ground ginger
- 1 tsp. ground coriander
- 1/2 tsp red pepper flakes
- 3 tbsp. low-sodium soy sauce
- 2 tbsp. honey
- 1 tbsp. lime juice
- 1 tbsp. green curry paste
- Optional: chopped peanuts for topping

Instructions:
1. Combine curry paste, honey, lime juice, soy sauce, and spices. Leave for now.
2. Drizzle sesame oil on a frying pan placed over medium heat. Cook chicken until well done. Transfer to a plate.
3. Add a drizzle of sesame oil and cook Egg Beaters.
4. Transfer to another plate when done.
5. In the same pan, add some sesame oil to cook the carrots, mushrooms, garlic, and pepper and onion blend.
6. Put chicken and egg back in the pan, and stir to combine.
7. Add zucchini noodles and cook until they soften.
8. Put in the sauce mixture, stir together, and cook for 5 more minutes.
9. Serve hot and sprinkle peanuts on top.

Chicken Broth

Ingredients:
- 1 chicken carcass from a leftover roast chicken or bones
- 2 cloves of garlic
- water
- Optional: carrot or parsnip tops, leftover vegetable peelings, and herbs

Instructions:
1. Cover chicken bones with water, whether cooking in a large stockpot, a pressure cooker, or a slow cooker.
2. For the slow cooker, cook on high for 4 hours.
3. For the pressure cooker, set it to cook for an hour.
4. For the stockpot, set it on a low simmer for 3 to 4 hours.
5. Once the time is up, strain the liquid from the broth through a sieve into a large bowl or container.
6. Discard the bones and garlic.
7. Keep the liquid, and pour it into a container.

Kale Fried Rice

Ingredients:
- 2 tbsp. coconut oil
- 2 whole eggs
- 2 large garlic cloves, minced
- 3 large green onions, thinly sliced
- 1 cup of carrots, cut into matchsticks
- 1 cup of Brussels sprouts, diced

1 medium bunch of kale, ribs removed and the leaves shredded
- 2 cups brown rice, cooked and cooled
- 1/4 tsp. Himalayan salt
- 1/4 cup of lemon balm leaves, diced
- 3/4 cups of shredded coconut, unsweetened variety
- fresh cilantro, for garnishing

Instructions:
1. Heat up a teaspoon of oil in a large skillet over medium-high heat.
2. Pour in the egg mixture.
3. Cook the eggs while occasionally stirring.
4. Remove from the pan and set aside.
5. Pour another teaspoon of coconut oil into the pan, along with Brussels sprouts, carrots, garlic, and green onions.
6. Stir every now and then until the vegetables look tender.
7. Add kale and salt.
8. Remove from the pan and put them into where the egg is.
9. Put the remaining coconut oil into the pan. Add in coconut flakes, stirring frequently
10. Add rice and stir it in.
11. Add the egg and vegetable mixture to the pan, as well as the lemon balm leaves.
12. Stir to combine and heat through.
13. Transfer to a serving bowl and garnish with fresh cilantro.
14. Serve and enjoy.

Stir-Fried Cabbage and Apples

Ingredients:
- 1 shallot, thinly sliced
- 1/2 apple, cut into cubes
- 1/4 savoy cabbage, sliced thinly into strips
- 3–4 radishes, sliced thinly
- 1/2–1 tsp. coconut oil
- salt, to taste

Instructions:
1. Pour some coconut oil into a wok.
2. Add shallot and cook until translucent.
3. Add the cabbage, radish, and apples to the wok.
4. Stir-fry for about 5 minutes. Don't overcook.
5. Add salt to taste.
6. Serve while warm.

Chicken Stir Fry

Ingredients:
- 1 tbsp. coconut oil
- 2 chicken breasts, cubed
- 1 red bell pepper, diced
- 1 cup broccoli florets
- 1 large sweet potato, shredded or spiralized
- 2 tbsp. parsley, chopped
- 1 tbsp. sesame seeds
- 1 lime, wedged

For the Turmeric Sauce:
- 1/2 can coconut milk
- 1 tbsp. almond butter
- 2 cloves garlic, minced
- 1 lime juiced
- 1 tsp. turmeric
- 1 tsp. sea salt
- 1/2 tsp. ginger powder, add more to taste
- 1/2 tsp. pepper

Instructions:
1. In a large skillet or wok placed on medium-high heat, pour in the coconut oil.
.2 Add chicken breasts and cook for 3-4 minutes per side
3. Add bell pepper, broccoli, and sweet potato noodles. Stir for 2-3 minutes.
4. While the chicken is cooking, whisk together the ingredients for the sauce.
5. Toss the mix with your spoon or tongs for 2-3 minutes.
6. Taste and adjust seasonings to your liking.
7. Top with parsley and sesame seeds.
8. Serve with lime wedges.

CONCLUSION

Histamine intolerance is a condition in which the body has difficulty breaking down and eliminating histamines. Symptoms of histamine intolerance can vary, but common signs include headaches, nausea, flushing, congestion, and skin irritation. The primary treatment for this condition is avoidance of foods high in histamines and adopting a low-histamine diet.

Following a low-histamine diet can be challenging but also beneficial to those who suffer from histamine intolerance. The key is to identify and avoid foods that are high in histamines or that cause an increased release of histamines into the body. For this reason, it's important to be aware of food triggers that could trigger symptoms. Additionally, foods full of probiotics such as yogurt or kefir may help reduce symptoms by promoting healthy gut bacteria which may aid in digestion and elimination of substances like histamines more effectively.

It's important to remember that each patient has different dietary needs when following a low-histamine diet as everyone reacts differently to specific types of foods as well as certain levels of histamines present in food. Therefore, it's best to speak with your doctor or qualified nutritionist about creating a diet plan tailored specifically for you based on your individual health needs and symptoms.

The goal is to maintain a balance between eating minimally processed foods while still avoiding high amounts of histamines within those foods. Eating plenty of fresh vegetables and fruits, nuts, legumes and small amounts of meat or fish are some options for maintaining nutrition while reducing potential sources for digestive issues associated with histamine intolerance.

Additionally, simple modifications to recipes can help reduce histamines or make them more suitable for your diet needs. Examples of this include substituting kombucha for vinegar in a salad dressing or baking with almond milk instead of regular milk. With some practice and dedication, it is possible to incorporate flavorful meals into a low-histamine diet plan.

FAQ

What is histamine intolerance?
Histamine intolerance is a condition characterized by symptoms such as headache, hives, abdominal pain, and diarrhea that are triggered by the consumption of foods that contain high levels of histamine. The condition is caused by an imbalance between the levels of histamine and diamine oxidase (an enzyme that breaks down histamine) in the body.

What are the symptoms of histamine intolerance?
The symptoms of histamine intolerance can vary from person to person, but they typically include headaches, hives, abdominal pain, and diarrhea. Some people may also experience nausea, vomiting, and difficulty breathing.

What foods should be avoided if you have histamine intolerance?
Several foods should be avoided if you have histamine intolerance, including aged cheese, fermented foods, cured meats, alcohol, and certain fruits and vegetables. A full list of foods to avoid can be found here:

What is the difference between a low-histamine diet and a histamine-free diet?
A low-histamine diet is a diet that includes only low levels of

histamine-containing foods. A histamine-free diet is a diet that eliminates all sources of histamine.

How long does it take for symptoms of histamine intolerance to appear?
Symptoms of histamine intolerance typically appear within minutes to hours after consuming food that contains high levels of histamine.

Is there a cure for histamine intolerance?
There is no cure for histamine intolerance, but symptoms can be managed by following a low-histamine or histamine-free diet.

Can Histamines be eliminated from the body?
No, Histamines cannot be eliminated from the body but they can be broken down by an enzyme called diamine oxidase (DAO).

What causes an imbalance of Histamines in the body?
There are many possible causes of an imbalance of Histamines in the body including gut dysbiosis, leaky gut syndrome, genetic factors, and certain medications.

How is Histamine Intolerance diagnosed?
A diagnosis of Histamine Intolerance is typically made based on symptoms and medical history. If necessary, blood tests or skin prick tests may also be used to confirm the diagnosis.

Are there any risks associated with following a low-histamine diet?
Yes, there are some risks associated with following a low-histamine diet including nutrient deficiencies and social isolation. However, these risks can be minimized by working with a registered dietitian or nutritionist to ensure that your diet is still balanced and meeting your nutritional needs.

REFERENCES AND HELPFUL LINKS

Burkhart, A. (2021, April 22). The low histamine diet: What is it and does it work? Amy Burkhart, MD, RD. https://theceliacmd.com/the-low-histamine-diet-what-is-it-and-does-it-work/.

Contributors, W. E. (n.d.). Foods high in histamine. WebMD. Retrieved March 2, 2023, from https://www.webmd.com/diet/foods-high-in-histamine.

Fowler, P. (n.d.). Histamines: What they do, and how they can overreact. WebMD. Retrieved March 2, 2023, from https://www.webmd.com/allergies/what-are-histamines.

Histamine intolerance: Causes, symptoms, and diagnosis. (2018, August 13). Healthline. https://www.healthline.com/health/histamine-intolerance.

Low histamine diet: Foods to eat and to avoid. (2020, June 11). https://www.medicalnewstoday.com/articles/low-histamine-diet.

Medlineplus: Histamine: the stuff allergies are made of.

(n.d.). Retrieved March 2, 2023, from https://medlineplus.gov/medlineplus-videos/histamine-the-stuff-allergies-are-made-of/.

What is a low-histamine diet? (n.d.). BBC Good Food. Retrieved March 2, 2023, from https://www.bbcgoodfood.com/howto/guide/what-low-histamine-diet.

Printed in Great Britain
by Amazon